THE ULTIMATE GUIDE TO HAIR CARE WITH ESSENTIAL OILS

Contents

Introduction

When it comes to achieving luscious, healthy locks of hair, essential oils have emerged as a popular and effective choice for hair care enthusiasts. These potent, aromatic oils are derived from various plant sources and have been cherished for their numerous therapeutic properties for centuries. In recent years, their application in hair care routines has gained significant attention, and for good reason. This comprehensive guide is your key to understanding why essential oils are a valuable addition to your hair care regimen and how to make the most of their natural benefits.

Why Essential Oils for Hair Care?

The allure of essential oils for hair care lies in their multifaceted approach to achieving and maintaining beautiful, vibrant hair. Here's why these oils have become a preferred choice for many:

1. **Natural and Chemical-Free:** Essential oils are derived from plant extracts, making them a natural alternative to commercial hair products loaded with chemicals and synthetic ingredients.

This natural approach reduces the risk of adverse reactions and long-term damage to your hair.

2. **Nourishment for Your Scalp:** The foundation of healthy hair is a healthy scalp. Essential oils are known for their ability to nourish the scalp, promoting optimal conditions for hair growth. They can help balance oil production, combat dandruff, and soothe irritation.

3. **Stimulate Hair Growth:** Certain essential oils have been studied for their potential to stimulate hair follicles and encourage new hair growth. If you are struggling with hair thinning or want to boost the volume of your locks, specific oils can be incredibly beneficial.

4. **Strengthens and Conditions:** Essential oils are rich in vitamins, antioxidants, and fatty acids that can fortify your hair shafts, making them less prone to breakage and split ends. They also add shine and softness to your locks.

5. **Aromatherapy Benefits:** Beyond their physical advantages, essential oils offer aromatherapeutic benefits. The invigorating scents can uplift your mood, reduce stress, and create a calming atmosphere during your hair care routines.

6. **Customizable Solutions:** Essential oils come in a wide variety, each with its unique properties and benefits. This means you can customize your hair care routine to address your specific needs, whether you have dry, oily, curly, or straight hair.

7. **Cost-Effective:** While high-quality essential oils may seem pricey upfront, they are concentrated and require only a few drops per use. This makes them a cost-effective choice compared to many commercial hair products.

8. **Environmental Consciousness:** Using essential oils in your hair care routine can align with environmentally conscious choices, as many commercial hair products contain harsh chemicals that may harm aquatic ecosystems when they are washed down the drain.

How to Use This Guide

Now that we have established why essential oils are worth exploring for your hair care, let us discuss how to navigate this guide to make the most of your journey to healthier, more radiant hair.

Chapter Structure: This guide is divided into chapters, each addressing specific aspects of essential oils for hair care. You will find information on understanding your hair type and common hair problems, as well as recommendations for essential oils tailored to different needs. Also included is a practical DIY hair care recipes and tips for incorporating essential oils into your routine.

Safety Precautions: Before diving into the world of essential oils, it is crucial to be aware of safety precautions. Essential oils are potent and should be handled with care. We will provide you with essential information on how to use these oils safely and what to watch out for to avoid any adverse reactions.

DIY Hair Care Recipes: In the "DIY Hair Care Recipes" chapter, you'll discover a treasure trove of natural hair care recipes that you can easily prepare at home. From homemade shampoos and conditioners to specialized scalp treatments and hair growth serums, these recipes will allow you to take control of your hair care routine.

Incorporating Essential Oils: Essential oils can be used in various ways to achieve the best results for your hair. In this section, we will guide you on how to incorporate essential oils into your daily, weekly, and monthly hair care routines. Whether you are looking for a quick boost or a more intensive treatment, we've got you covered.

Tips for Healthy Hair: Achieving and maintaining healthy hair goes beyond just using essential oils. We will share valuable tips on nutrition, lifestyle factors, and proper styling techniques that can complement your essential oil-based hair care routine.

Quality Matters: Not all essential oils are created equal. In "Essential Oil Brands and Quality," we will help you choose the right essential oils and guide you on where to purchase them. Ensuring you have high-quality oils is essential for reaping the full benefits.

Frequently Asked Questions: We've compiled a list of frequently asked questions related to essential oils for hair care. This section will provide answers to common queries, dispelling any doubts or uncertainties you may have.

Conclusion: In the concluding chapter, we'll recap the key takeaways from this guide, emphasizing the importance of embracing the journey to beautiful hair through the natural power of essential oils.

Appendices: Lastly, you will find useful appendices that serve as quick references, a glossary of terms for those new to essential oils, and a list of additional resources and references for further exploration.

Are you ready to embark on your journey to healthier, more beautiful hair with the help of essential oils? Let's dive in and discover the natural wonders that await you!

Chapter 1: Understanding Your Hair

Before we delve into the world of essential oils for hair care, it is essential to have a solid understanding of your hair. Hair is as diverse as the individuals it adorns, and recognizing your hair type, texture, and common problems is the first step toward tailoring a successful hair care routine. In this chapter, we will explore the intricacies of hair types and textures, common hair problems, and how essential oils can play a vital role in addressing these issues.

Hair Types and Texture

Hair is not a one-size-fits-all entity. Just as our skin and body types vary, so does our hair. Understanding your unique hair type and texture is fundamental to selecting the right essential oils and hair care practices for your specific needs.

Hair Types

Hair types are generally classified into four main categories:

1. **Straight Hair:** Straight hair typically lies flat against the scalp and lacks natural curls or waves. It tends to be smooth and sleek, but it can also be prone to looking flat and lifeless.

2. **Wavy Hair:** Wavy hair falls somewhere between straight and curly. It has gentle, loose waves that add texture and volume to the hair. Wavy hair can be quite versatile and respond well to various hair care routines.

3. **Curly Hair:** Curly hair is characterized by well-defined curls or spirals. It often has a natural bounce and can range from loose curls to tight coils. Curly hair tends to be more prone to frizz and dryness.

4. **Kinky or Coily Hair:** This hair type features tightly coiled or zigzag-shaped strands. It is common among people of African descent. Kinky hair can be delicate and prone to breakage if not properly cared for, but it can also be incredibly resilient and beautiful when given the right attention.

Hair Texture

Hair texture refers to the thickness or diameter of individual hair strands. It is typically categorized into three main types:

1. **Fine Hair:** Fine hair has a small diameter, making it appear thinner and more delicate. It can be prone to looking flat and may lack volume.

2. **Medium Hair:** Medium hair falls in between fine and coarse. It is a common hair texture and tends to be more manageable and versatile.

3. **Coarse air:** Coarse hair has a larger diameter, giving it a thicker and more robust appearance. It can be prone to frizz and may require more moisture to maintain its health and luster.

Understanding both your hair type and texture is essential because it determines how your hair responds to different hair care products and treatments. For instance, individuals with curly or coily hair may struggle with dryness and frizz, while those with fine hair might battle with flatness and lack of volume. Essential oils can be particularly helpful in addressing these unique challenges.

Common Hair Problems

No matter your hair type or texture, various common hair problems can affect anyone. Recognizing these issues is crucial to developing an effective hair care routine that incorporates essential oils.

1. **Dry and Dehydrated Hair:** Dry hair lacks moisture and can become brittle, leading to breakage and split ends. It often appears dull and lifeless.

2. **Oily Hair**: Excess oil production can make hair look greasy and weighed down. It can also contribute to scalp issues like dandruff.

3. **Dandruff and Scalp Issues:** Dandruff is characterized by flaky, itchy, or irritated scalp. It can be caused by various factors, including dryness, excess oil, or fungal overgrowth.

4. **Hair Loss and Thinning:** Hair loss can be due to genetic factors, hormonal changes, stress, or poor hair care practices. Thinning hair can lead to reduced volume and density.

5. **Split Ends and Breakage:** Split ends occur when the hair shaft splits into two or more strands. Breakage can happen due to various factors, including excessive heat styling and chemical treatments.

6. **Frizz and Flyaways:** Frizzy hair is often a result of dryness and lack of control over the hair cuticle. Flyaways are those unruly, stray strands that refuse to stay in place.

The Role of Essential Oils

Now that we have explored the diversity of hair types and common problems, let us delve into the exciting world of essential oils and how they can be your hair's best friend.

Nourishing the Scalp: Essential oils are renowned for their ability to nourish the scalp. A healthy scalp is the foundation of healthy hair growth. Many essential oils, such as lavender, rosemary, and tea tree oil, possess soothing and moisturizing properties that can alleviate dryness and irritation. Massaging these oils into your scalp can stimulate blood flow, promote relaxation, and create an optimal environment for hair growth.

Balancing Oil Production: If you struggle with oily hair, essential oils like lemon, peppermint, and cedarwood can help regulate sebum production. These oils have astringent properties that can reduce excess oil on the scalp and keep your hair looking fresh for longer periods.

Stimulating Hair Growth: One of the most exciting benefits of essential oils is their potential to stimulate hair growth. Oils like rosemary, peppermint, and lavender have been studied for their ability to promote hair follicle activity and encourage new hair growth. These oils work by increasing blood circulation to the scalp and providing essential nutrients to the hair follicles.

Fortifying and Conditioning: Essential oils are rich in vitamins, antioxidants, and fatty acids that can strengthen and condition your hair. They help repair damage, reduce split ends, and add shine and softness. Oils like argan, jojoba, and coconut are renowned for their deep conditioning properties.

Combatting Dandruff: If you are dealing with dandruff or other scalp issues, essential oils like tea tree oil, eucalyptus, and lavender can come to your rescue. These oils have antifungal and antibacterial properties that can address the root causes of dandruff and provide relief from itching and flaking.

Reducing Hair Loss and Breakage: Essential oils can help reduce hair loss and breakage by strengthening the hair shafts. Oils like cedarwood, thyme, and clary sage can improve hair's resistance to damage and minimize hair loss.

Controlling Frizz and Flyaways: Frizzy hair can benefit from essential oils like argan and jojoba, which provide deep hydration and help seal the hair cuticle. This results in smoother, more manageable hair that is less prone to frizz and flyaways.

In this guide, we will explore the specific essential oils that are best suited to address these common hair problems and how to incorporate them into your hair care routine. Whether your goal is to achieve luscious, long locks, or simply maintain a healthy and manageable mane, essential oils offer a natural and holistic approach to hair care that can yield impressive results.

Understanding your hair type, texture, and the specific challenges you face is the first step towards creating a customized hair care regimen that harnesses the power of essential oils. By the end of this guide, you will have the knowledge and tools needed to embark on a hair care journey that not only transforms your locks but also elevates your overall well-being.

Chapter 2: Getting Started with Essential Oils

Now that you have gained insight into your unique hair type, texture, and common hair problems, it is time to dive into the world of essential oils for hair care. This chapter serves as a comprehensive guide to help you get started on your journey towards healthier, more beautiful hair. We will cover the basics, including an introduction to essential oils, safety precautions, the importance of carrier oils, and a selection of essential oils specifically beneficial for hair.

Introduction to Essential Oils

Essential oils are highly concentrated, aromatic compounds extracted from various parts of plants, including flowers, leaves, stems, and roots. These oils are often referred to as the "essence" of the plant, as they capture the plant's distinct scent and therapeutic properties.

One of the remarkable aspects of essential oils is their versatility. They have been used for centuries in traditional medicine, aromatherapy, skincare, and, of course, hair care. The power of essential oils lies in their ability to address a wide range of physical and emotional concerns.

Key Characteristics of Essential Oils for Hair Care:

1. **Aromatherapeutic Benefits:** Many essential oils offer mood-enhancing and stress-reducing benefits. Incorporating them into your hair care routine can create a soothing and enjoyable experience.

2. **Natural and Pure:** To reap the full benefits, it is crucial to use high-quality, pure essential oils. Look for oils that are labelled as 100% pure and therapeutic grade.

3. **Highly Concentrated:** Essential oils are potent, and only a few drops are usually needed for each application. This makes them cost-effective in the long run.

4. **Varied Scents:** Essential oils come in a wide array of scents, from floral and citrusy to earthy and woody. You can choose oils that resonate with your personal preferences.

Safety Precautions

While essential oils offer numerous benefits, they are potent substances that should be handled with care. Here are some essential safety precautions to keep in mind when using essential oils for hair care:

1. **Dilution:** Essential oils are highly concentrated and can be too strong for direct application to the skin or hair. Always dilute them with a carrier oil (discussed below) before use.

2. **Patch Test:** Before using any new essential oil, perform a patch test on a small area of your skin to check for allergic reactions or sensitivity.

3. **Keep Out of Reach of Children:** Essential oils should be stored out of reach of children and pets. Ingestion or improper use can be harmful.

4. **Phototoxicity:** Some citrus essential oils, like bergamot and lime, can make your skin more sensitive to sunlight. Avoid sun exposure for 12-24 hours after applying these oils.

5. **Pregnancy and Medical Conditions:** If you are pregnant, nursing, or have underlying medical conditions, consult with a healthcare professional before using essential oils.

6. **Quality Matters:** Invest in high-quality, pure essential oils from reputable brands. Cheap or synthetic oils may not deliver the same benefits and can be potentially harmful.

Carrier Oils: Your Base

Carrier oils are non-volatile, fatty oils derived from seeds, nuts, or vegetables. They serve as a base for diluting essential oils before application to the skin or hair. Carrier oils are essential for safe and effective use of essential oils in hair care.

Key Functions of Carrier Oils:

1. **Dilution:** Carrier oils dilute the concentration of essential oils, reducing the risk of skin or scalp irritation.

2. **Nourishment:** They provide additional nourishment to your hair and scalp, as they are rich in vitamins, antioxidants, and fatty acids.

3. **Stability:** Carrier oils help stabilize and extend the shelf life of essential oils.

4. **Ease of Application:** Carrier oils make it easier to apply essential oils evenly to your hair and scalp.

Popular Carrier Oils for Hair Care:

1. **Jojoba Oil:** Jojoba oil closely resembles the natural sebum produced by our skin and scalp. It is an excellent choice for all hair types and can help balance oil production.

2. **Coconut Oil:** Coconut oil is highly moisturizing and can penetrate the hair shaft, making it a popular choice for deep conditioning treatments.

3. **Argan Oil:** Known as "liquid gold," argan oil is rich in vitamin E and antioxidants. It helps improve hair's elasticity and adds shine.

4. **Sweet Almond Oil:** Sweet almond oil is lightweight and nourishing, making it suitable for all hair types. It can reduce hair breakage and promote a healthy scalp.

5. **Grapeseed Oil:** Grapeseed oil is a light, non-greasy oil that can help control frizz and add shine to the hair.

6. **Olive Oil:** Olive oil is a versatile option for both hair and scalp. It's moisturizing and can help with dandruff and dryness.

Essential Oils for Hair

Now that you have a good understanding of essential oils and carrier oils, let us explore a selection of essential oils that are particularly beneficial for various hair types and common hair problems.

1. **Lavender Oil:** Lavender oil is known for its calming scent and soothing properties. It is excellent for promoting relaxation during your hair care routine. Lavender oil can also help balance oil production on the scalp and support hair growth.

2. **Rosemary Oil:** Rosemary oil is a powerhouse for hair care. It is been studied for its potential to stimulate hair follicles and promote hair growth. It is particularly useful for those dealing with hair loss or thinning.

3. **Peppermint Oil:** Peppermint oil has a refreshing and invigorating scent. It is known for its ability to increase blood circulation to the scalp, which can promote hair growth and reduce dandruff.

4. **Tea Tree Oil:** Tea tree oil is highly effective for addressing dandruff and scalp issues. Its antifungal and antibacterial properties can help soothe an irritated scalp.

5. **Cedarwood Oil:** Cedarwood oil can help balance oil production on the scalp, making it beneficial for those with oily hair. It also has a warm, woody scent.

6. **Lemon Oil:** Lemon oil is a natural astringent that can help control excess oil on the scalp. It adds a fresh, citrusy scent to your hair care routine.

7. **Chamomile Oil:** Chamomile oil is gentle and soothing. It can help reduce scalp irritation and is suitable for those with sensitive skin.

8. **Ylang Ylang Oil:** Ylang ylang oil has a sweet and floral scent. It is used to promote hair growth and reduce hair breakage.

9. **Clary Sage Oil:** Clary sage oil is known for its ability to regulate oil production on the scalp. It has a herbal, earthy scent.

10. **Geranium Oil:** Geranium oil can help balance oil production and promote hair growth. It has a pleasant floral scent.

By understanding the properties of these oils and how they relate to your unique hair type

and concerns, you will be well-equipped to
create personalized hair care recipes that bring
out the best in your locks

.

Understanding your hair type is the foundation of a successful hair care routine. Each hair type comes with its unique set of challenges and requirements, and essential oils can play a pivotal role in addressing these needs. In this chapter, we will explore how essential oils can be tailored to cater to various hair types, from dry and curly to oily and straight. Discover the right essential oils for your hair type to achieve healthy, beautiful locks.

Oils for Dry Hair

Dry hair is characterized by a lack of moisture and often appears dull, rough, and prone to frizz. It may be caused by factors such as excessive heat styling, overwashing, exposure to harsh weather conditions, or genetics. Essential oils can provide much-needed hydration and nourishment to dry hair, restoring its natural shine and vitality.

Recommended Essential Oils for Dry Hair:

1. **Jojoba Oil:** Jojoba oil closely mimics the natural sebum produced by the scalp, making it an excellent choice for dry hair. It provides deep hydration, reduces frizz, and leaves hair soft and manageable.

2. **Argan Oil:** Known as "liquid gold," argan oil is rich in vitamin E and essential fatty acids. It helps repair damage, adds shine, and restores moisture to dry hair.

3. **Coconut Oil:** Coconut oil is a popular choice for deep conditioning dry hair. It penetrates the hair shaft to provide intense hydration and improve overall hair health.

4. **Avocado Oil:** Avocado oil is packed with vitamins, including vitamin E and B, which promote hair growth and strengthen hair strands. It's an excellent choice for dry and brittle hair.

5. **Rosehip Oil:** Rosehip oil is rich in antioxidants and can help repair and rejuvenate dry hair. It's especially useful for restoring shine and managing frizz.

6. **Ylang Ylang Oil:** Ylang ylang oil not only has a lovely floral scent but also helps balance sebum production on the scalp. This can prevent

dryness and promote healthier, more moisturized hair.

To use essential oils for dry hair, you can add a few drops of your chosen oil to a carrier oil, such as jojoba or argan oil, and apply it to your hair and scalp. Leave it on for a few hours or overnight, then shampoo and condition as usual. Regular use can help combat dryness and improve the overall texture of your hair.

Oils for Oily Hair

Oily hair is characterized by excess sebum production, making it appear greasy and weighed down. Oily hair can be caused by hormonal imbalances, genetics, or simply overactive sebaceous glands. Essential oils with astringent properties can help control excess oil production and leave your hair looking fresh and clean.

Recommended Essential Oils for Oily Hair:

1. **Lemon Oil:** Lemon oil is a natural astringent that helps regulate oil production on the scalp. It adds a fresh, citrusy scent to your hair and can combat greasiness.

2. **Tea Tree Oil:** Tea tree oil has potent antifungal and antibacterial properties, making it effective in addressing scalp issues that can lead to excess oil production. It also has a refreshing scent.

3. **Peppermint Oil:** Peppermint oil stimulates blood circulation in the scalp, which can help reduce oiliness. Its invigorating scent is also a bonus.

4. **Cedarwood Oil:** Cedarwood oil can help balance sebum production and is suitable for those with an oily scalp. Its warm, woody scent is grounding and comforting.

5. **Lavender Oil:** Lavender oil not only has a calming aroma but also helps balance oil production. It is a versatile oil that can benefit both your hair and your overall well-being.

To use essential oils for oily hair, dilute a few drops of your chosen oil in a carrier oil like jojoba or grapeseed oil. Apply the mixture to your scalp and massage it in, then leave it on for at least 30 minutes before washing your hair. This process can help control excess oil and maintain a fresh, clean feel.

Oils for Normal Hair

If you have normal hair, consider yourself fortunate! Normal hair falls in the middle of the dry-oily spectrum, and it typically does not require as much attention as extreme hair types. However, using essential oils can enhance the health and appearance of your hair, keeping it in excellent condition.

Recommended Essential Oils for Normal Hair:

1. **Rosemary Oil:** Rosemary oil is a versatile option that supports hair growth and strengthens hair strands. It can help maintain the health and vitality of normal hair.

2. **Chamomile Oil:** Chamomile oil is gentle and soothing, making it an excellent choice for normal hair. It can enhance shine and maintain a healthy scalp.

3. **Geranium Oil:** Geranium oil can help balance oil production, making it suitable for normal hair that occasionally leans towards dryness or oiliness. Its floral scent is pleasing and calming.

4. **Clary Sage Oil:** Clary sage oil is known for its ability to regulate sebum production. It is a well-rounded option for normal hair care.

To use essential oils for normal hair, dilute a few drops in a carrier oil and apply the mixture to your hair and scalp. You can use this as a pre-shampoo treatment or add a few drops to your regular shampoo and conditioner. This will help maintain the health and beauty of your normal hair, keeping it in optimal condition.

Oils for Curly Hair

Curly hair is known for its natural bounce and texture, but it can also be prone to dryness, frizz, and tangling. The right essential oils can help enhance the curl pattern, reduce frizz, and keep your curls looking their best.

Recommended Essential Oils for Curly Hair:

1. **Argan Oil:** Argan oil is a go-to choice for curly hair. It is highly moisturizing and helps define curls while reducing frizz.

2. **Shea Butter Oil:** Shea butter oil is rich and nourishing, making it perfect for maintaining moisture in curly hair. It helps with detangling and adds shine.

3. **Coconut Oil:** Coconut oil can penetrate the hair shaft, providing deep hydration to curly

locks. It is a popular choice for deep conditioning treatments.

4. **Jojoba Oil:** Jojoba oil is lightweight and helps control frizz in curly hair. It can also define curls and maintain their shape.

5. **Lavender Oil:** Lavender oil has a soothing aroma and can help balance the scalp's oil production, making it suitable for curly hair types.

To use essential oils for curly hair, mix a few drops with a carrier oil and apply it to your hair, focusing on the ends and any areas prone to frizz. You can also add a few drops to your leave-in conditioner or styling products to enhance curl definition.

Oils for Straight Hair

Straight hair often has a smooth and sleek appearance, but it can still face challenges such as flatness and lack of volume. Essential oils can provide the necessary nourishment and support to maintain healthy, glossy straight hair.

Recommended Essential Oils for Straight Hair:

1. **Rosehip Oil:** Rosehip oil is lightweight and absorbs quickly, making it suitable for straight hair. It adds shine and helps maintain hair health.

2. **Lemon Oil:** Lemon oil is a natural astringent that can help control oiliness in straight hair. Its fresh scent is invigorating.

3. **Ylang Ylang Oil:** Ylang ylang oil can add a floral fragrance and promote hair growth. It's a lovely addition to straight hair care routines.

4. **Peppermint Oil:** Peppermint oil stimulates blood flow to the scalp, which can help maintain hair health and add volume to straight hair.

To use essential oils for straight hair, dilute a few drops in a carrier oil and apply it to your hair, paying attention to the ends and any areas that need extra care. You can also add a few drops to your regular shampoo and conditioner to infuse your hair care routine with the benefits of essential oils.

Incorporating essential oils into your hair care routine can be a game-changer, regardless of your hair type. Whether you are looking to combat dryness, control oiliness, enhance curls, or add volume to straight locks, there is an essential oil that can help you achieve your hair goals. Experiment with different oils, and do not be afraid to mix and match to create customized hair care solutions that work best for your unique hair type and preferences. In the next chapters, we will delve deeper into DIY hair care recipes and how to make the most of these essential oils for specific hair concerns.

Chapter 4: Essential Oils for Common Hair Problems

Every hair type, no matter how diverse, can experience common hair problems. Whether you are dealing with dandruff, hair loss, split ends, or frizz, essential oils offer a natural and effective solution to address these concerns. In this chapter, we will explore how to use essential oils to tackle these common hair issues and restore your hair's health and vitality.

Dandruff and Scalp Issues

Dandruff is a common scalp condition characterized by the shedding of flaky skin. It can be caused by factors such as dry skin, excess oil, fungal overgrowth, or sensitivity to hair care products. Essential oils with antimicrobial, antifungal, and soothing properties can help combat dandruff and alleviate scalp irritation.

Recommended Essential Oils for Dandruff and Scalp Issues:

1. **Tea Tree Oil:** Tea tree oil is a potent antifungal and antibacterial oil that can effectively address the root causes of dandruff. It soothes scalp irritation and helps maintain a healthy scalp.

2. **Lavender Oil:** Lavender oil has both calming and antimicrobial properties, making it an excellent choice for reducing scalp irritation and promoting a balanced scalp environment.

3. **Rosemary Oil:** Rosemary oil stimulates blood circulation in the scalp, which can help improve scalp health and reduce dandruff. It also supports hair growth.

4. **Peppermint Oil:** Peppermint oil has a cooling effect on the scalp and helps relieve itching. Its antimicrobial properties can also address the underlying causes of dandruff.

To use essential oils for dandruff and scalp issues, mix a few drops with a carrier oil (such as jojoba or coconut oil) and massage the mixture into your scalp. Leave it on for at least 30 minutes before washing your hair. Regular use can help reduce dandruff and maintain a healthy, flake-free scalp.

Hair Loss and Thinning

Hair loss and thinning hair can be caused by various factors, including genetics, hormonal changes, stress, and poor hair care practices. Essential oils known for their ability to stimulate hair follicles and improve hair thickness can be valuable in addressing hair loss and thinning.

Recommended Essential Oils for Hair Loss and Thinning:

1. **Rosemary Oil:** Rosemary oil is a powerful hair growth stimulant. It increases blood circulation to the scalp, promoting hair follicle activity and hair growth.

2. **Lavender Oil:** Lavender oil not only has a pleasant aroma but also helps improve hair thickness and promote hair growth.

3. **Cedarwood Oil:** Cedarwood oil can help reduce hair loss by balancing oil production and promoting a healthy scalp environment.

4. **Peppermint Oil:** Peppermint oil's cooling effect can stimulate blood flow to the scalp and encourage hair growth.

5. **Thyme Oil:** Thyme oil has been shown to promote hair growth and reduce hair loss when applied to the scalp.

To use essential oils for hair loss and thinning, add a few drops to a carrier oil and massage the mixture into your scalp. Leave it on for a few hours or overnight before washing your hair. Consistency is key when using essential oils to address hair loss, so make it a regular part of your routine.

Split Ends and Breakage

Split ends and hair breakage can occur due to various factors, including excessive heat styling, chemical treatments, and inadequate hair care practices. Essential oils with nourishing and strengthening properties can help reduce split ends and breakage.

Recommended Essential Oils for Split Ends and Breakage:

1. **Argan Oil:** Argan oil is rich in vitamin E and essential fatty acids. It helps repair split ends and strengthen hair, reducing breakage.

2. **Jojoba Oil:** Jojoba oil's lightweight texture makes it ideal for preventing split ends. It hydrates the hair shaft and adds shine.

3. **Sweet Almond Oil:** Sweet almond oil is rich in vitamins and antioxidants that nourish the hair, reducing the risk of breakage.

4. **Coconut Oil:** Coconut oil penetrates the hair shaft, providing deep conditioning and reducing split ends. It is especially beneficial for damaged hair.

To use essential oils for split ends and breakage, apply a few drops of your chosen oil to the ends of your hair. You can also use these oils as a pre-shampoo treatment by applying them to your hair and leaving them on for at least 30 minutes before washing.

Frizz and Flyaways

Frizz and flyaways are common hair annoyances, especially in humid climates or for those with naturally curly or wavy hair. Essential oils with moisturizing and smoothing properties can help tame frizz and keep your hair looking sleek.

Recommended Essential Oils for Frizz and Flyaways:

1. **Argan Oil:** Argan oil is a go-to choice for controlling frizz and adding shine. It tames unruly hair and keeps it manageable.

2. **Jojoba Oil:** Jojoba oil helps control frizz and provides a protective barrier to prevent moisture loss in the hair.

3. **Shea Butter Oil:** Shea butter oil is rich and moisturizing, making it effective at taming frizz and flyaways.

4. **Coconut Oil:** Coconut oil can help reduce frizz by adding moisture to the hair shaft and preventing excess moisture from getting in.

5. **Rosehip Oil:** Rosehip oil is lightweight and helps smooth the hair cuticle, reducing frizz and improving hair texture.

To use essential oils for frizz and flyaways, apply a few drops to your palms and run them through your hair, focusing on the areas prone to frizz. You can also add a few drops to your regular conditioner or use them as a styling product to keep your hair sleek and frizz-free.

Incorporating essential oils into your hair care routine to address common hair problems is a natural and effective way to maintain the health and beauty of your hair. Whether you are dealing with dandruff, hair loss, split ends, or frizz, there is an essential oil solution that can help you achieve the hair you desire.

 Experiment with different oils and techniques to find the best approach for your specific concerns, and enjoy the transformation of your locks as you harness the power of nature's remedies.

Chapter 5: DIY Hair Care Recipes

Embarking on a journey to healthier, more beautiful hair does not always require a trip to the store. With the right ingredients and a little creativity, you can create your own DIY hair care products that cater to your specific needs. In this chapter, we will explore a variety of homemade recipes, including shampoos, conditioners, hair masks, scalp treatments, and hair growth serums, all enriched with the goodness of essential oils.

Homemade Shampoos

Creating your own homemade shampoo allows you to control the ingredients and tailor the formula to your hair type and concerns. These DIY shampoo recipes incorporate essential oils that provide nourishment, balance, and a delightful scent to your hair cleansing routine.

1. Nourishing Honey and Lavender Shampoo:

Ingredients:

- 1/4 cup liquid castile soap

- 2 tablespoons raw honey

- 10 drops lavender essential oil

- 5 drops rosemary essential oil

- 5 drops tea tree essential oil

Instructions:

1. In a mixing bowl, combine the liquid castile soap and raw honey.

2. Add the lavender, rosemary, and tea tree essential oils and stir well to blend.

3. Transfer the mixture to a squeeze bottle or pump dispenser for easy use.

How to Use:

Wet your hair thoroughly and apply a small amount of the shampoo to your scalp and hair. Massage gently to create a lather, then rinse with warm water. Follow with a homemade conditioner or your preferred conditioner.

2. Soothing Aloe Vera and Peppermint Shampoo:

Ingredients:

- 1/4 cup aloe vera gel

- 1/4 cup liquid castile soap

- 10 drops peppermint essential oil

- 5 drops chamomile essential oil

- 5 drops lavender essential oil

Instructions:

1. In a mixing bowl, combine the aloe vera gel and liquid castile soap.

2. Add the peppermint, chamomile, and lavender essential oils and mix thoroughly.

3. Pour the mixture into a squeeze bottle or pump dispenser for convenient use.

How to Use:

Apply a small amount of the shampoo to wet hair, focusing on the scalp. Massage gently to create a lather, then rinse thoroughly with warm water. Follow with a homemade conditioner or your preferred conditioner.

Conditioners and Hair Masks

Homemade conditioners and hair masks are excellent for providing deep hydration and nourishment to your hair. They can help improve hair texture, reduce frizz, and enhance shine. Here are some DIY recipes that incorporate essential oils for added benefits.

1. Moisturizing Coconut and Lavender Conditioner:

Ingredients:

- 1/2 cup coconut oil

- 10 drops lavender essential oil

- 5 drops rosemary essential oil

Instructions:

1. In a microwave-safe bowl, melt the coconut oil until it becomes a liquid (if it is not already).

2. Allow the melted coconut oil to cool slightly, then add the lavender and rosemary essential oils. Mix well.

3. Transfer the mixture to a clean, empty conditioner bottle or jar.

How to Use:

After shampooing your hair, apply a small amount of the conditioner to the lengths and ends of your hair. Leave it on for 5-10 minutes, then rinse thoroughly with warm water.

2. Avocado and Honey Hair Mask:

Ingredients:

- 1 ripe avocado

- 2 tablespoons raw honey

- 10 drops argan oil

Instructions:

1. Mash the ripe avocado in a bowl until it becomes a smooth paste.

2. Add the raw honey and argan oil, then mix until all ingredients are well combined.

3. Apply the mask to clean, damp hair, focusing on the ends. Leave it on for 20-30 minutes.

4. Rinse the mask out with warm water and follow with a mild shampoo if necessary.

Scalp Treatments

A healthy scalp is the foundation for healthy hair growth. These DIY scalp treatments infused with essential oils can help address scalp issues and promote optimal hair growth conditions.

1. Tea Tree and Coconut Oil Scalp Treatment:

Ingredients:

- 2 tablespoons coconut oil

- 5 drops tea tree essential oil

- 5 drops rosemary essential oil

Instructions:

1. In a small bowl, melt the coconut oil until it's in liquid form.

2. Allow the oil to cool slightly, then add the tea tree and rosemary essential oils. Mix well.

3. Using your fingertips, massage the mixture into your scalp in gentle, circular motions.

4. Leave the treatment on for at least 30 minutes or overnight for deep penetration.

5. Wash your hair with a mild shampoo and conditioner.

2. Aloe Vera and Lavender Scalp Soothing Serum:

Ingredients:

- 1/4 cup aloe vera gel

- 10 drops lavender essential oil

- 5 drops chamomile essential oil

Instructions:

1. In a small bowl, combine the aloe vera gel, lavender essential oil, and chamomile essential oil. Mix well.

2. Transfer the serum to a clean, empty dropper bottle for easy application.

How to Use:

Apply a few drops of the serum directly to your scalp and massage it in using your fingertips. Leave it on without rinsing for a soothing scalp treatment. Use as needed.

Hair Growth Serums

If you are looking to boost hair growth and improve the overall health of your hair, these DIY hair growth serums enriched with essential oils can be a valuable addition to your routine.

1. Rosemary and Jojoba Hair Growth Serum:

Ingredients:

- 1/4 cup jojoba oil

- 10 drops rosemary essential oil

- 5 drops cedarwood essential oil

Instructions:

1. In a clean, empty dropper bottle, combine the jojoba oil, rosemary essential oil, and cedarwood essential oil. Shake well to blend.

How to Use:

Apply a few drops of the serum directly to your scalp and gently massage it in. Leave it on without rinsing. For best results, use this serum regularly to stimulate hair follicles and promote healthy hair growth.

2. Castor Oil and Peppermint Hair Growth Serum:

Ingredients:

- 1/4 cup castor oil

- 10 drops peppermint essential oil

- 5 drops lavender essential oil

Instructions:

1. In a clean, empty dropper bottle, combine the castor oil, peppermint essential oil, and lavender essential oil. Shake well to mix.

How to Use:

Apply a few drops of the serum to your scalp and massage it in using gentle, circular motions. Leave it on without rinsing. This serum can help improve circulation to the scalp and stimulate hair growth when used regularly.

Creating your own DIY hair care products with essential oils allows you to take control of the ingredients you use and personalize your hair care routine. Whether you are making your own shampoo, conditioner, hair mask, scalp treatment, or hair growth serum, you can infuse them with the natural benefits of essential oils to achieve the hair of your dreams. Experiment with these recipes, and do not hesitate to tailor them to your specific needs and preferences. Your hair will thank you for the extra care and attention it receives from these homemade concoctions.

Chapter 6: Incorporating Essential Oils into Your Hair Care Routine

Now that you have a collection of essential oil-infused DIY hair care products at your disposal, it is essential to understand how to incorporate them seamlessly into your hair care routine. In this chapter, we will explore various strategies for integrating essential oils into your daily, weekly, and monthly hair care rituals, ensuring that your locks receive the love and nourishment they deserve.

Daily Hair Care

Your daily hair care routine sets the foundation for healthy and beautiful hair. By incorporating essential oils into your daily regimen, you can address specific concerns and maintain the overall health of your hair.

1. Essential Oil-Enriched Shampoo and Conditioner:

Start your day with a gentle, essential oil-infused shampoo and conditioner. Choose a combination that aligns with your hair type and concerns. Apply the shampoo to wet hair, massaging it into your scalp for a refreshing and cleansing experience. Follow up with the conditioner to nourish and detangle your locks. Rinse thoroughly with water.

2. Lightweight Essential Oil Serum:

For a daily boost of hair health, create a lightweight essential oil serum. Mix a few drops of your preferred essential oil (such as lavender or rosemary) with a carrier oil like jojoba or argan oil. Apply a small amount to your hair ends and lengths to keep them hydrated and protected throughout the day.

3. Hair Perfume with Essential Oils:

If you love the idea of fragrant hair, consider creating a hair perfume infused with essential oils. Combine your favourite essential oils with a neutral carrier oil or alcohol in a small spray bottle. Give your hair a gentle mist for a pleasing aroma that lasts all day.

Weekly Hair Care Rituals

Incorporating essential oils into your weekly hair care rituals allows for deeper nourishment and targeted treatments. These rituals can help address specific concerns and maintain the overall health of your hair.

1. Deep Conditioning Hair Mask:

Once a week, treat your hair to a deep conditioning mask infused with essential oils. Choose a mask recipe that aligns with your hair type and concerns. Apply the mask to clean, damp hair, focusing on the lengths and ends. Leave it on for the recommended time, usually 20-30 minutes. Rinse thoroughly with warm water and enjoy the softness and shine.

2. Scalp Massage with Essential Oils:

Consider incorporating a weekly scalp massage using essential oils to stimulate blood circulation and promote a healthy scalp. Create a scalp treatment with essential oils like rosemary, lavender, or tea tree mixed with a carrier oil. Gently massage the mixture into your scalp using circular motions. Leave it on for at least 30 minutes before shampooing.

3. Essential Oil-Infused Hair Rinse:

After shampooing and conditioning your hair, give it a final rinse with an essential oil-infused water mixture. Prepare a solution by adding a few drops of your chosen essential oil (such as rosemary or chamomile) to a bowl of lukewarm water. Pour it over your hair as a final rinse to lock in the benefits of essential oils and leave your hair smelling delightful.

Monthly Treatments

Monthly treatments provide an opportunity for more intensive care and addressing specific hair concerns. By incorporating essential oils into your monthly routine, you can achieve remarkable results over time.

1. Hair Growth Serum Application:

If you are focused on hair growth, use a hair growth serum infused with essential oils once a month. Apply the serum directly to your scalp and massage the serum in using gentle, circular motions. Leave it on without rinsing overnight or for at least a few hours before washing your hair.

2. Clarifying Essential Oil Treatment:

Once a month, treat your hair to a clarifying treatment with essential oils to remove buildup from styling products and hard water minerals. Mix a few drops of a clarifying essential oil like lemon or tea tree with a mild, sulfate-free shampoo. Use this mixture to cleanse your hair, focusing on the roots and scalp, and rinse thoroughly.

3. Restorative Hair Mask:

Give your hair a monthly dose of restoration with a deep hair mask that incorporates essential oils. These masks can help repair damage, reduce split ends, and improve hair texture. Choose a mask recipe suitable for your hair type and concerns and follow the application instructions provided.

Additional Tips for Incorporating Essential Oils:

1. **Customization is Key:** Tailor your essential oil choices to your specific hair type, concerns, and preferences. Experiment with different oils and blends to find what works best for you.

2. **Patch Testing:** Before using any new essential oil or product, perform a patch test on a small area of your skin to ensure you do not have any adverse reactions or allergies.

3. **Storage:** Store your essential oils in a cool, dark place away from direct sunlight and heat to preserve their potency.

4. **Quality Matters:** Invest in high-quality, 100% pure essential oils from reputable brands to ensure you get the best results.

5. **Consistency:** Consistency is key when using essential oils for hair care. Stick to your routine and be patient; it may take time to see significant improvements.

6. **Safety Precautions:** Always follow safety guidelines and recommendations for essential oil use, including proper dilution, especially when applying them directly to the skin or scalp.

By incorporating essential oils into your daily, weekly, and monthly hair care rituals, you can create a holistic and personalized approach to hair care. These natural remedies can help address specific concerns, maintain hair health, and promote a luxurious and aromatic hair care experience. Enjoy the journey of nurturing your hair with the power of essential oils and watch your locks flourish with vitality and beauty.

Chapter 7: Tips for Healthy Hair

Having a luxurious mane of healthy hair is a desire shared by many. While essential oils and DIY treatments can certainly play a significant role in achieving and maintaining beautiful hair, there are several other factors that contribute to the overall health and appearance of your locks. In this chapter, we will explore essential tips and practices for promoting healthy hair from the inside out, considering nutrition, lifestyle factors, and styling and heat protection.

Nutrition and Diet

1. **Balanced Diet:** Your hair's health starts from within, so it is essential to maintain a balanced diet. Incorporate a variety of nutrients, including protein, vitamins, and minerals, to support hair growth and strength. Foods rich in biotin (such as eggs), iron (like spinach), and omega-3 fatty acids (found in fatty fish like salmon) are particularly beneficial for hair health.

2. **Stay Hydrated:** Proper hydration is crucial for hair health. Drinking enough water helps keep

your hair and scalp moisturized, reducing the risk of dryness and brittleness.

3. **Protein Intake:** Hair is primarily made of a protein called keratin, so it is essential to consume an adequate amount of protein in your diet. Include sources like lean meats, beans, and dairy products to ensure your hair gets the protein it needs.

4. **Vitamins and Supplements:** If your diet lacks essential vitamins and minerals, consider taking supplements, but only under the guidance of a healthcare professional. Biotin, vitamin D, and iron supplements can be particularly beneficial for hair health.

5. **Avoid Crash Diets:** Extreme diets or rapid weight loss can lead to hair loss. It is important to maintain a healthy, gradual weight loss if needed, to minimize the risk of hair damage.

Lifestyle Factors

1. **Manage Stress**: Chronic stress can lead to hair loss and other scalp issues. Practice stress management techniques like meditation, yoga, or deep breathing exercises to keep stress levels in check.

2. **Regular Exercise:** Physical activity promotes healthy circulation, including to the scalp. Exercise also helps reduce stress, which can indirectly benefit your hair.

3. **Adequate Sleep:** Your body uses sleep as a time for repair and regeneration, including hair growth. Aim for 7-9 hours of quality sleep each night to support healthy hair.

4. **Gentle Hair Care:** Be gentle with your hair to avoid unnecessary breakage. Use a wide-toothed comb to detangle wet hair, and avoid pulling or tying your hair too tightly.

5. **Reduce Heat Styling:** Limit the use of heat styling tools such as straighteners and curling irons, as excessive heat can damage the hair shaft and lead to breakage. When you do use them, apply a heat protectant spray first.6. Protect Your Hair from the Sun: Prolonged sun exposure can weaken hair and cause color fading. Wear a hat or use hair products with UV protection when spending time in the sun.

7. **Avoid Overwashing**: Washing your hair daily can strip it of its natural oils, leading to dryness and potential damage. Try to limit hair washing to 2-3 times a week, or as needed based on your hair type and activities.

8. **Use Gentle Hair Products:** Choose shampoos and conditioners that are sulfate-free and suitable for your hair type. Harsh chemicals can strip your hair of its natural oils and lead to dryness.

Styling and Heat Protection

1. **Heat Protection Products:** Always use a heat protectant spray or serum before using heat styling tools. These products create a barrier that shields your hair from the high temperatures.

2. **Cooling Off Period:** Allow your hair to cool down after using heat styling tools before styling or brushing it further. This can help set the style and reduce the risk of damage.

3. **Adjust Heat Settings:** Use the lowest effective heat setting on your styling tools to achieve the desired results. High temperatures can damage hair quickly.

4. **Limit Heat Usage:** Whenever possible, opt for heatless hairstyles like braids, buns, or air-drying. This reduces the frequency of heat styling, minimizing potential damage.

5. **Regular Trims:** Schedule regular hair trims every 6-8 weeks to remove split ends and prevent them from traveling up the hair shaft, causing more damage.

6. **Avoid Tight Hairstyles:** Tight ponytails, buns, or braids can cause stress on the hair shaft and lead to breakage or hair loss. Opt for looser hairstyles and avoid constant tension on the hair.

7. **Protective Hairstyles:** Consider protective hairstyles like buns or twists that keep your hair tucked away and shielded from environmental damage.

8. **Silk or Satin Pillowcases:** Sleeping on silk or satin pillowcases can reduce friction and help prevent hair breakage and frizz. Cotton pillowcases can cause hair to rub and tangle.

9. **Cold Water Rinse:** After washing your hair, finish with a cold water rinse. This can help close the hair cuticles, making your hair smoother and shinier.

10. **Chemical Treatments:** If you are considering chemical treatments like colouring or perming, be sure to go to a professional who uses quality products and follows proper procedures to minimize damage.

Remember that achieving and maintaining healthy hair is a journey that requires patience and consistency. By incorporating these tips into your daily routine and paying attention to your diet, lifestyle, and hair care practices, you can promote the health and beauty of your hair from the inside out. Additionally, combining these practices with the use of essential oils and DIY treatments as discussed in previous chapters can help you achieve and maintain the vibrant and healthy hair you desire.

Chapter 8: Essential Oil Brands and Quality

When it comes to harnessing the power of essential oils for your hair care routine, choosing the right essential oil brands and ensuring their quality and purity are paramount. In this chapter, we will explore the factors to consider when selecting essential oils, where to buy them, and how to determine their quality and purity.

Choosing the Right Essential Oils

Selecting the right essential oils for your hair care needs is crucial to achieving the best results. Here are some considerations to keep in mind:

1. **Hair Type and Concerns:** Identify your hair type and specific concerns. Different essential oils offer various benefits, so choose oils that align with your hair's unique needs. For example, lavender is known for its calming and soothing properties, while rosemary is excellent for stimulating hair growth.

2. **Quality and Purity:** Opt for high-quality, 100% pure essential oils from reputable brands. Ensure that the oils have not been diluted with carrier oils or synthetic fragrances, as this can diminish their effectiveness.

3. **Scent Preference:** Essential oils come in a wide range of scents, from floral and herbal to citrus and woody. Select oils with scents that you enjoy, as the aroma can enhance your hair care experience.

4. **Blending Options:** Consider whether you want to blend essential oils to create custom hair care solutions. Some essential oils pair well together and can address multiple concerns simultaneously.

5. **Allergies and Sensitivities:** If you have known allergies or sensitivities to certain essential oils, be cautious and avoid those oils in your hair care routine.

Where to Buy Essential Oils

Finding a reliable source for essential oils is crucial to ensuring their quality and effectiveness. Here are some options for where to purchase essential oils:

1. **Reputable Brands:** Purchase essential oils from well-established and reputable brands known for their commitment to quality. Look for brands that provide transparency about their sourcing and testing processes.

2. **Specialty Stores:** Many health food stores and specialty shops carry a selection of essential oils. Be sure to inquire about the source and quality of the oils before making a purchase.

3. **Online Retailers:** There are numerous online retailers that sell essential oils. Look for websites that provide detailed information about each oil, including its source, extraction method, and purity. Customer reviews can also offer insights into the quality of the oils.

4. **Aromatherapy Suppliers:** Suppliers that cater to aromatherapists and holistic practitioners often carry high-quality essential oils. These suppliers may offer a broader selection of oils and accessories.

5. **Direct Sales Companies**: Some essential oil brands operate through direct sales representatives. While these companies can provide access to quality oils, it is essential to research the specific brand and ensure that the representative is knowledgeable about the products.

6. **Local Distilleries:** If you have access to local distilleries or farms that produce essential oils, consider purchasing directly from them. This can provide assurance about the sourcing and purity of the oils.

Quality and Purity

Determining the quality and purity of essential oils is crucial to their effectiveness and safety. Here are some factors to consider when evaluating essential oils:

1. **Botanical Name:** Each essential oil should have its botanical name on the label. This ensures that you are getting the correct plant species, as different species can have varying properties.

2. **Purity:** Look for essential oils labelled as "100% pure" or "pure essential oil." Avoid oils labelled as "fragrance oils" or "perfume oils," as these may contain synthetic ingredients.

3. **Testing and Certification:** Reputable brands often subject their essential oils to third-party testing to verify their purity and quality. Look for oils that have been tested and certified by organizations such as the International Organization for Standardization (ISO) or the

Association for the Advancement of Sustainable Aromatherapy (AASA).

4. **Sourcing and Origin:** Learn about the source and origin of the essential oils. High-quality oils are often sourced from regions known for producing specific plant varieties. Ethical and sustainable sourcing practices are also important.

5. **Extraction Method:** The method used to extract essential oils can impact their quality. Common extraction methods include steam distillation, cold-pressing, and CO_2 extraction. Research the preferred extraction method for a particular oil.

6. **Storage and Packaging:** Essential oils are sensitive to light, heat, and air, which can cause them to deteriorate. Ensure that the oils are packaged in dark glass bottles with tight-sealing caps and stored in a cool, dark place.

7. **Price:** While price alone is not a definitive indicator of quality, exceptionally low prices may be a red flag. High-quality essential oils require significant quantities of plant material for extraction, making them more expensive than low-quality alternatives.

8. **Smell Test:** A genuine essential oil should have a strong, natural aroma that corresponds to the plant it was derived from. If the scent is weak or unnatural, it may indicate adulteration.

9. **Safety Information:** Reputable brands provide safety information, including any potential contraindications or precautions associated with specific oils. Always follow these guidelines to ensure safe use.

10. **Customer Reviews:** Reading reviews and testimonials from other customers can provide insights into the quality and effectiveness of essential oils from a particular brand.

It is important to note that essential oils are highly concentrated and potent substances. When using them for hair care or any other purpose, always follow recommended dilution guidelines and safety precautions.

Incorporating essential oils into your hair care routine can be a transformative experience, provided you select high-quality oils from reputable sources. By carefully choosing the right essential oils, where you purchase them, and ensuring their quality and purity, you can enjoy the full benefits of these natural remedies and achieve healthier, more beautiful hair.

Chapter 9: Frequently Asked Questions

As you delve into the world of essential oils and their application for hair care, you may encounter a range of questions and uncertainties. This chapter is designed to address some of the most frequently asked questions regarding essential oils and their role in maintaining healthy and beautiful hair.

1. Are essential oils safe for all hair types?

Essential oils can be safe and beneficial for various hair types, including dry, oily, curly, straight, and more. However, it is essential to choose the right oils for your specific hair concerns and to use them in appropriate dilutions. Always perform a patch test before applying essential oils directly to your scalp or hair to ensure you do not experience adverse reactions or allergies.

2. Are Essential Oils Safe to Use on the Scalp?

Essential oils can be safe for use on the scalp when used correctly. However, they are highly concentrated and should always be diluted with a carrier oil before applying directly to the scalp to avoid potential skin irritation or sensitivity. It's also essential to perform a patch test to check for any adverse reactions before using a new essential oil.

3. What Are Essential Oils, and How Are They Extracted?

Essential oils are highly concentrated, aromatic liquids extracted from various parts of plants, including leaves, flowers, stems, roots, and seeds. They are obtained through a process known as distillation, which involves the following steps:

1. **Harvesting:** The plant material is carefully harvested at the peak of its aromatic potency.

2. **Steam Distillation:** The most common method of extraction is steam distillation. Steam is passed through the plant material, causing it to release its essential oil. The steam and oil vapor are then condensed and separated, with the essential oil collecting on top.

3. **Cold Pressing:** Some essential oils, such as citrus oils (e.g., orange, lemon, and grapefruit), are extracted through a process called cold pressing. This method involves mechanically pressing the oil from the plant's peel.

4. **CO2 Extraction:** CO2 extraction is a more modern method that uses carbon dioxide as a solvent to extract essential oils. It yields oils with minimal heat exposure, preserving their quality.

5. **Solvent Extraction:** Less commonly, some essential oils are obtained through solvent extraction, which involves using chemical solvents to dissolve the oil from the plant material.

The resulting essential oils are highly concentrated and should be used with care and proper dilution.

4. How should I dilute essential oils for hair care?

Diluting essential oils is crucial to ensure their safe use. A general guideline for dilution is to add 1-2% essential oil to a carrier oil, such as jojoba, coconut, or argan oil. For example, if you have 1 ounce (30 mL) of carrier oil, you can add 6-12 drops of essential oil. However, the exact dilution may vary depending on the essential oil and your specific needs. Be sure to research the recommended dilution rates for each oil and hair concern.

5. Can essential oils promote hair growth?

Some essential oils, such as rosemary, cedarwood, lavender, and peppermint, have been associated with promoting hair growth. These oils can stimulate blood circulation to the scalp, which, in turn, may support hair follicle activity and encourage hair growth. Remember that results may vary, and consistency in use is essential when using essential oils for hair growth.

6. How often should I use essential oils for hair care?

The frequency of using essential oils for hair care can vary based on your specific needs and goals. Daily use of essential oils in small quantities, such as in shampoos or leave-in treatments, is generally safe for most people. However, deep conditioning masks and intensive scalp treatments may only need to be done once a week or less frequently. Always follow the recommended usage guidelines provided for each essential oil and hair care product.

7. Can essential oils replace commercial hair care products?

While essential oils can be a valuable addition to your hair care routine, they are not a one-size-fits-all solution. Some commercial hair care products serve specific purposes, such as colour protection, hydration, or styling, that essential oils alone may not provide. You can integrate essential oils into your existing routine or create DIY alternatives, but it's essential to consider your individual hair care needs and preferences.

8. Are there any essential oils to avoid during pregnancy or while breastfeeding?

Certain essential oils should be used with caution during pregnancy and breastfeeding due to their potential effects on hormones and the developing fetus or infant. Oils such as clary sage, juniper berry, and rosemary should be avoided during pregnancy. It is advisable to consult with a healthcare professional or aromatherapist for personalized guidance on essential oil use during these periods.

9. Can I ingest essential oils for hair benefits?

Ingesting essential oils is generally not recommended unless under the guidance of a qualified healthcare professional or aromatherapist. Essential oils are highly concentrated and can be toxic when consumed inappropriately. It is safer to use essential oils topically or aromatically for hair care.

10. How can I minimize the scent of essential oils in my hair?

If you find the scent of essential oils too strong in your hair, you can dilute the oils more in your hair care products or choose essential oils with milder aromas. Additionally, consider using fewer drops of essential oil when creating your DIY hair care recipes. Over time, you may also become more accustomed to the scent.

11. Can I use essential oils on coloured or chemically treated hair?

Essential oils can typically be used on coloured or chemically treated hair without causing significant issues. However, if you have specific concerns, such as maintaining colour longevity, you can choose essential oils that are gentle and nourishing, like lavender or chamomile. Always perform a patch test before using essential oils on coloured or chemically treated hair to ensure there is no adverse reaction.

12. Can Essential Oils Help with Dandruff and Scalp Issues?

Yes, many essential oils have antimicrobial, antifungal, and soothing properties that can help address dandruff and scalp issues. Tea tree oil, lavender oil, rosemary oil, and peppermint oil are examples of essential oils that can effectively combat dandruff, reduce scalp irritation, and promote a healthy scalp environment.

13. What Carrier Oils Are Best for Mixing with Essential Oils?

Carrier oils are used to dilute essential oils and help spread them evenly on the skin or scalp. The choice of carrier oil can vary based on personal preference and hair type, but some commonly used carrier oils for hair care include:

- Jojoba Oil: Suitable for all hair types, jojoba oil closely resembles the natural oils produced by the scalp and is easily absorbed.

- Coconut Oil: Ideal for dry and damaged hair, coconut oil provides deep conditioning and nourishment.

- Argan Oil: Known for its high vitamin E content, argan oil is excellent for adding shine and reducing frizz.

- Sweet Almond Oil: A lightweight option that works well for most hair types, sweet almond oil is rich in vitamins and antioxidants.

- Olive Oil: Another versatile option, olive oil can help moisturize and strengthen hair.

- Grapeseed Oil: Suitable for fine or thin hair, grapeseed oil is lightweight and won't weigh down the hair.

The choice of carrier oil can also depend on personal preference, scent, and the desired outcome.

14. Can Essential Oils Be Used in Shampoos and Conditioners?

Yes, you can incorporate essential oils into your shampoo and conditioner by adding a few drops to the bottles. Ensure that you mix them well before use. This allows you to enjoy the benefits of essential oils with every wash.

15. Can I Blend Essential Oils Together?

Yes, blending essential oils can be a powerful way to create custom solutions for your hair care needs. However, it is crucial to research and follow recommended dilution ratios and safety guidelines for each essential oil. Not all essential oils blend well together, so some experimentation may be required to find the right combinations.

16. How Long Does It Take to See Results with Essential Oils for Hair Care?

A: The time it takes to see results with essential oils for hair care can vary from person to person and depends on factors such as the specific concern being addressed, the frequency of use, and individual hair growth rates. In some cases, you may notice improvements in hair texture and condition within a few weeks, while hair growth results may take several months of consistent use.

17. Can Essential Oils Cause Allergic Reactions?

Yes, some individuals may be sensitive or allergic to certain essential oils. Before using a new essential oil, perform a patch test by applying a diluted solution to a small area of skin to check for any adverse reactions. If you experience redness, itching, or irritation, discontinue use.

Chapter 10: Conclusion

Congratulations on completing this comprehensive guide to using essential oils for hair care! Throughout this book, you have gained insights into the world of essential oils, learned how to select the right oils for your hair type and concerns, and discovered various DIY recipes and techniques to promote healthier and more beautiful hair. In this concluding chapter, we will recap the key takeaways from your journey into the realm of essential oil-infused hair care and encourage you to continue embracing this path to stunning locks.

Recap of Key Takeaways

1. Understanding Essential Oils:

   - Essential oils are highly concentrated plant extracts that offer a wide range of benefits for hair care.

   - They are derived from various parts of plants, such as leaves, flowers, bark, and roots, through methods like steam distillation and cold-pressing.

2. Choosing the Right Essential Oils:

   - Select essential oils that align with your hair type, concerns, and preferences.

   - Be mindful of the quality and purity of essential oils, opting for 100% pure oils from reputable brands.

   - Always perform a patch test before applying essential oils to your scalp or hair to avoid adverse reactions.

3. Using Essential Oils for Different Hair Types:

   - Essential oils can benefit all hair types, including dry, oily, curly, and straight hair.

   - Customize your essential oil blends and hair care products to address your specific needs.

4. Addressing Common Hair Problems:

   - Essential oils can help combat common hair issues, such as dandruff, hair loss, split ends, and frizz.

   - Incorporate essential oils into your weekly and monthly hair care rituals to see long-term improvements.

5. DIY Hair Care Recipes:

   - Explore a variety of DIY hair care recipes, including shampoos, conditioners, hair masks, scalp treatments, and hair growth serums.

   - Personalize these recipes to cater to your unique hair needs and preferences.

6. Incorporating Essential Oils into Your Routine:

   - Integrate essential oils into your daily, weekly, and monthly hair care routines for consistent benefits.

   - Be patient and consistent in your use of essential oils, as it may take time to see significant improvements.

7. Maintaining Healthy Hair:

   - Pay attention to your nutrition and diet, ensuring you consume a balanced intake of protein, vitamins, and minerals.

   - Manage stress, prioritize exercise and sleep, and avoid harsh styling practices to maintain overall hair health.

   - Protect your hair from heat styling tools and minimize exposure to harmful UV rays.

8. Selecting High-Quality Essential Oils:

   - Purchase essential oils from reputable brands that prioritize quality, purity, and transparency.

   - Look for third-party testing and certifications to verify the authenticity of the oils.

Embracing the Journey to Beautiful Hair

Your journey to beautiful, healthy hair is ongoing, and incorporating essential oils into your hair care routine is just one aspect of this transformative process. Here are some final words of encouragement to help you continue on this path:

1. Be Patient and Consistent: Achieving and maintaining healthy hair takes time and consistency. Continue to use essential oils and other hair care practices regularly to see lasting results.

2. Stay Informed: The world of hair care and essential oils is constantly evolving. Stay informed about new research, products, and techniques that can enhance your hair care routine.

3. Tailor Your Approach: Your hair is unique, so don't be afraid to tailor your hair care routine to suit your individual needs. Experiment with different essential oil blends and treatments to find what works best for you.

4. Holistic Care: Remember that beautiful hair starts from the inside out. A balanced diet, stress management, and overall well-being play a significant role in the health of your hair.

5. Consult Professionals: If you have specific hair concerns or conditions, consider consulting with a dermatologist or trichologist for expert guidance. They can help diagnose and address underlying issues.

6. Share Your Knowledge: Share your newfound knowledge of essential oils and hair care with friends and family who may benefit from these natural remedies.

7. Celebrate Your Progress: Celebrate small victories along the way. Whether it's achieving your hair growth goals or simply enjoying the delightful aroma of your DIY hair products, every step forward is worth celebrating.

In conclusion, your journey to beautiful hair is a holistic and ongoing process that combines the power of essential oils with a balanced lifestyle and personalized care. By understanding the unique needs of your hair, selecting high-quality essential oils, and consistently embracing natural remedies, you can achieve and maintain the vibrant and healthy locks you desire. Continue to nurture your hair with love and attention, and enjoy the beauty that naturally unfolds on this path.

Appendices

In this section, you will find a collection of valuable resources and references to enhance your understanding of essential oils and their application in hair care. These appendices serve as handy tools to refer to throughout your journey towards healthier, more vibrant hair.

Appendix A: Essential Oil Quick Reference Guide

This quick reference guide provides a concise overview of commonly used essential oils for hair care, their benefits, and recommended uses. Use this guide as a handy reference when selecting oils for your specific hair type and concerns.

1. **Lavender Oil**

   - Benefits: Soothes scalp, promotes hair growth, adds shine.

   - Uses: Scalp massage, hair masks, aromatherapy.

2. **Rosemary Oil**

   - Benefits: Stimulates hair growth, improves circulation, strengthens hair.

   - Uses: Scalp massage, hair rinse, DIY shampoos.

3. **Tea Tree Oil**

   - Benefits: Treats dandruff, soothes scalp irritation, fights infections.

   - Uses: Dandruff treatments, scalp serums, anti-fungal blends.

4. **Peppermint Oil**

   - Benefits: Increases blood flow to scalp, invigorates hair follicles, adds shine.

   - Uses: Scalp massage, DIY hair growth treatments, refreshing sprays.

5. **Chamomile Oil**

   - Benefits: Soothes scalp, enhances hair color, conditions hair.

   - Uses: Hair rinses, DIY conditioners, aromatherapy.

6. **Cedarwood Oil**

   - Benefits: Stimulates hair follicles, reduces hair loss, balances oil production.

   - Uses: Scalp treatments, hair serums, DIY shampoos.

7. **Ylang Ylang Oil**

   - Benefits: Balances scalp oiliness, promotes healthy hair growth, adds shine.

   - Uses: Hair masks, scalp massages, aromatic blends.

8. **Clary Sage Oil**

   - Benefits: Regulates oil production, strengthens hair, promotes shine.

   - Uses: DIY hair care products, scalp treatments.

9. **Lemon Oil**

   - Benefits: Clarifies scalp, boosts shine, combats dandruff.

   - Uses: DIY shampoos, hair rinses, refreshing sprays.

10. **Geranium Oil**

   - Benefits: Balances oil production, adds shine, conditions hair.

   - Uses: DIY conditioners, hair masks, aromatherapy.

Appendix B: Glossary of Terms

This glossary provides definitions for key terms related to essential oils and hair care, helping you navigate the world of natural hair care with confidence.

1. **Carrier Oil:** A neutral, plant-based oil used to dilute essential oils for safe application on the skin or hair.

2. **Distillation:** The process of extracting essential oils from plant material using steam or water.

3. **Dilution:** Mixing essential oils with a carrier oil or another medium to reduce their concentration and minimize potential skin irritation.

4. **Patch Test:** A method of testing a small amount of diluted essential oil on a small area

of skin to check for allergic reactions or sensitivities.

5. **Steam Distillation:** A common method of essential oil extraction that uses steam to release the oils from plant material.

6. **Cold Pressing:** A method of extracting essential oils from citrus peels by mechanically pressing them.

7. **CO2 Extraction:** A modern method of extracting essential oils using carbon dioxide as a solvent.

8. **Antimicrobial:** Having the ability to inhibit or kill microorganisms like bacteria, fungi, and viruses.

9. **Aromatherapy:** The use of essential oils for therapeutic purposes, often through inhalation or topical application.

10. **Sulfate-Free:** Hair care products that do not contain sulfates, which can be harsh and drying to the hair.

Appendix C: Resources and References

This section provides a curated list of recommended resources, books, websites, and references for further exploration of essential oils, hair care, and related topics. These sources offer valuable information, recipes, and expert insights to support your journey towards healthier, more beautiful hair.

1. **Books:**

   - "The Complete Book of Essential Oils and Aromatherapy" by Valerie Ann Worwood

   - "The Essential Oils Handbook: All the Oils You Will Ever Need for Health, Vitality, and Well-Being" by Jennie Harding

2. **Websites and Blogs:**

   - [Aromaweb](https://www.aromaweb.com/): A comprehensive resource for information on essential oils, aromatherapy, and recipes.

   - [National Association for Holistic Aromatherapy (NAHA)](https://naha.org/): Provides education and resources on the safe and effective use of essential oils.

3. **Online Retailers:**

   - [Mountain Rose Herbs](https://www.mountainroseherbs.com/): Offers a wide range of high-quality, organic essential oils.

   - [Plant Therapy](https://www.planttherapy.com/): Known for their high-quality, affordable essential oils and blends.

4. **Scientific Journals:**

   - "Journal of Essential Oil Research": Publishes peer-reviewed research articles on essential oils and their applications.

   - "Phytotherapy Research": Covers research on herbal medicines, including essential oils.

5. **Hair Care Forums and Communities:**

   - [NaturallyCurly Forums](https://www.naturallycurly.com/curltalk/): A community for individuals with curly and natural hair, often discussing natural hair care methods.

6. **Safety and Usage Guides:**

   - [The Tisserand
Institute](https://tisserandinstitute.org/):
Provides evidence-based resources on essential
oil safety and usage.